Natural Skincare and Teenage Acne

Curing Skin Ailments Naturally

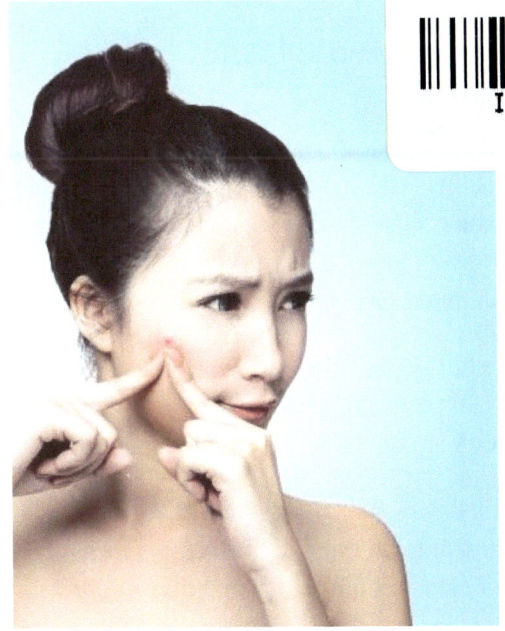

Dueep Jyot Singh

Healthy Living Series

Mendon Cottage Books

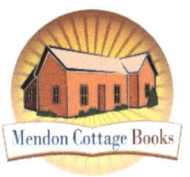

JD-Biz Publishing

Our books are available at

1. Amazon.com

2. Barnes and Noble

3. Itunes

4. Kobo

5. Smashwords

6. Google Play Books

Table of Contents

Introduction

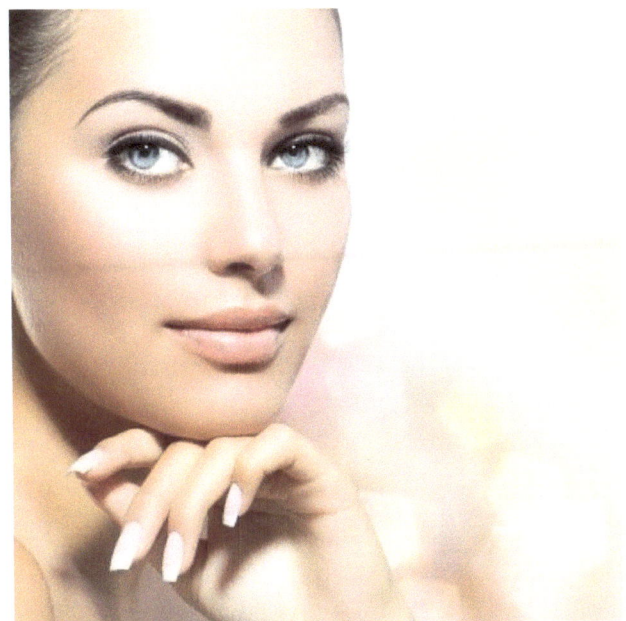

A beautiful, rare, perfect and healthy glowing skin is a thing of beauty, and a joy forever.

For millenniums, one of the main criteria of a beautiful and physically attractive person is considered to be the skin. A skin without any blemishes, ageless, without wrinkles, glowing, healthy, and with a luminosity is considered to be one of the top priorities of a health-conscious person.

Taking care of your skin is definitely not considered to be a narcissistic attitude. Instead, it shows that you intend to look good for your own self pride and ego. In many parts of the world, where I have been, I have seen plenty of women saying that they have not bothered looking after themselves, after a certain age, because people are going to say that they still want to hold onto their passing youth.

How absurd! In fact, these women are going to be appreciated even more, if the people around them show that they are well kept, well groomed, and take care of themselves, which includes hair, body, and skin.

This book is going to tell you all about how you can keep your face ageless, tackle teenage acne, and get rid of skin problems through natural remedies and cures.

Are Massages Necessary?

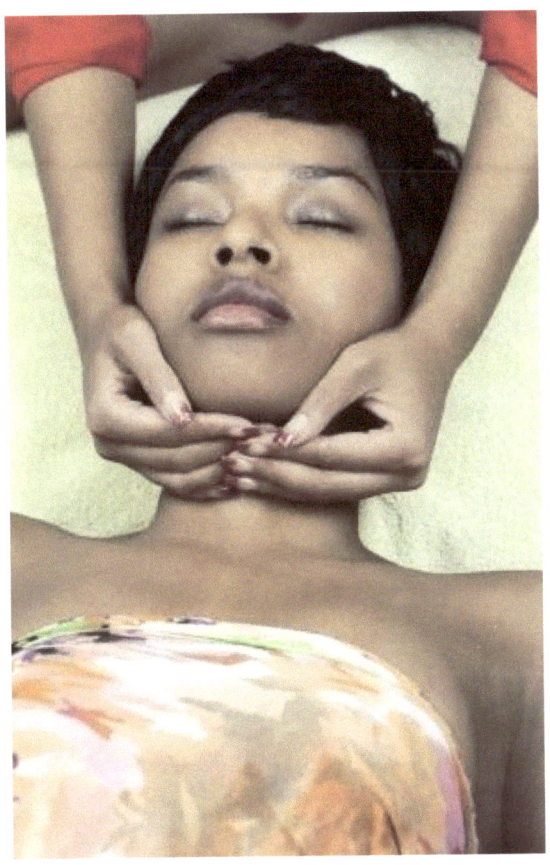

How many times have you just looked into a beauty salon, to see perfectly beautiful young ladies in their early 20s or even teenagers getting their faces massaged and interfered with chemical products? They intend to look more beautiful and that can only be done by very expensive chemical face packs, face massages, and face treatments. This has been told to them by their pet beauty saloon friend who welcomes them every 15 days to massage their faces with chemical-based creams.

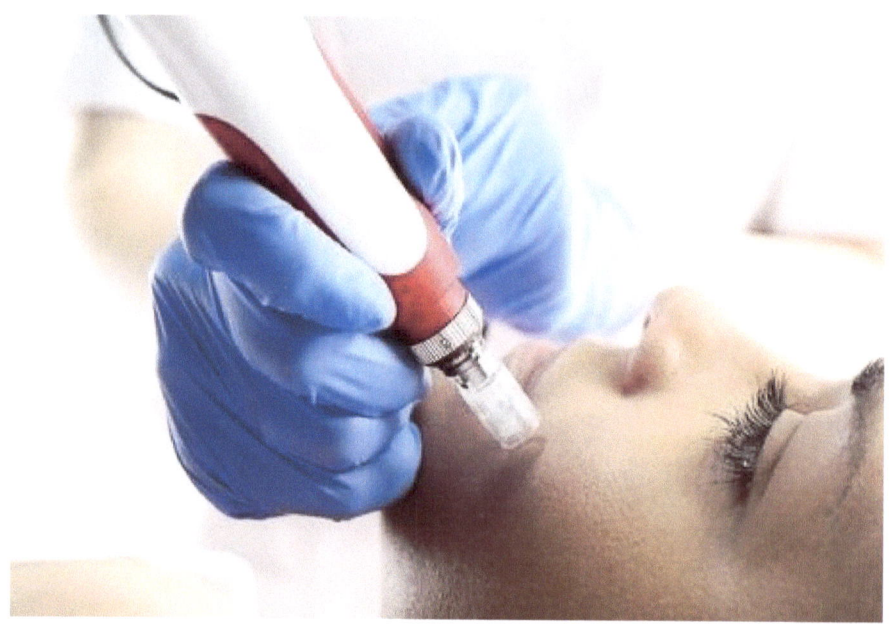

And the bill is really exorbitant. But these young girls are going to go home satisfied that they do not have a single wrinkle on their faces!

In fact, there are plenty of sites online, which teach you how to massage your own face right at home. However, it is not easier for you to do that, because the trouble happens to be that your arms are in the wrong position! A proper massage given to firm up sagging muscles and the contours of the face can only be done by someone who is standing behind you!

Try it out. You will give up after five minutes of pressure on your upper arms, trying to massage your face.

Nowadays, nearly every beauty saloon has a course of treatment where you can get your face reconditioned that is because there are so many rejuvenating facial packs along with herbal packs and other natural packs in the market that many of their clients demand the full treatment. But how useful is this treatment, you may ask?

Let me just give you an example. Just go into your kitchen, take some tomato pulp, at a little bit of cream to it, and a little bit of honey and one cube of ice to this mixture. Apply this mixture all over your face. Apart from your skin feeling really cold and tingly due to the ice, you are going to feel your skin feeling fresh and rejuvenated. Leave it on for 20 minutes. Then wash it off with warm water.

Now touch your skin. It feels really young looking, soft, moisturized, and plump.

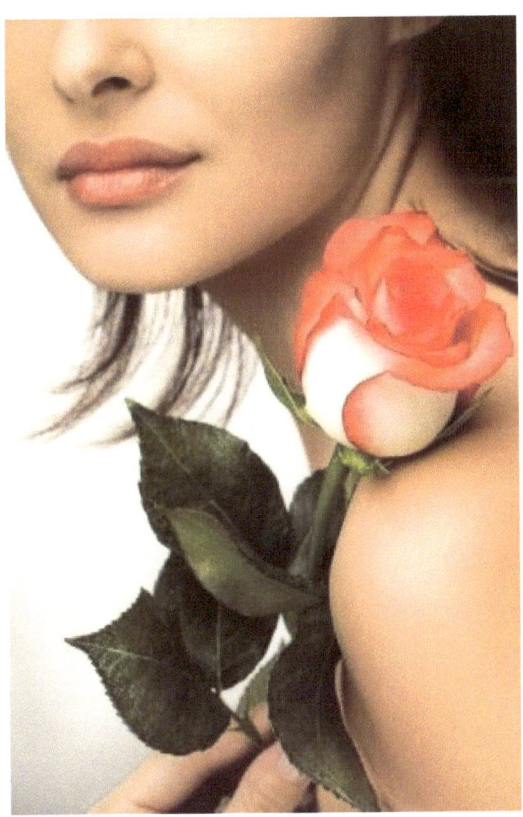

Psychologically, that is the same thing which has occurred, when you went to a beauty salon. Some herbs, lotions, potions, and creams were applied to your face. A professional pressed some pressure points, on your forehead, cheeks, at the back of your ears, under your chin and other pressure points, and you feel relaxed.

This treatment is going to take depending on what you want to get done. It can be anywhere from half an hour to more than four hours. In fact, in many beauty salons, you have to book ahead for the full day, to get a bridal beauty treatment done this facial treatment can take anywhere between 2 ½ - 3 hours, but then that appointment has been taken for this purpose.

These packages are normally going to consist of a facial massage, face packs to remove the sunburn, bleaching, removal of excess facial hair, and also the shaping of eyebrows at the very least.

Many people feel that they look brighter, cleaner, and freshly painted, when they come out after such a treatment. Of course, this treatment is just temporary. Sometimes it is drastic. It happened to me as well as my cousin.

My cousin suffered from a light coating of hair on her back, which made her very conscious. Nobody noticed it, especially when she was on the beach, but she being a beautiful young woman was conscious about something which she could not even see!

So she got a hair removal treatment done by one of the most expensive saloons in California. To her shock, her skin was burnt, and the treatment went all astray. Luckily, she was coming to India, where my grandmother treated those chemical burns with a mixture of milk, cream, and turmeric every evening. By the time she was ready to go back home to the USA, the burn marks were nearly gone.

You may say, that this is the one in a million chance, but when it happens twice in one family, it becomes a bit more than coincidence. It was my niece's wedding day and my cousin brother and sister-in-law told me to get really dolled up, where my brother was paying for the beauty treatment of all his sisters and cousins.

Naturally, I went in for the most expensive facial treatment which I had never tried before, but which was supposedly good enough to make my skin glow like gold and pearls.

It glowed literally and figuratively. It glowed so beautifully throughout the evening, that everybody complimented me on my beautiful "red and white" complexion! By the next morning, my whole skin had turned dark, because of chemical burns.

This happened in 2012. It is 2015 now and I am still trying to get rid of those chemical burns on my forehead and cheeks with natural remedies like aloe Vera and milk and turmeric, with tomato and lemon at night..

This is the reason why I request all my friends to keep away from beauty salons, with their chemical-based treatments. One of my aunts wanted to give me a gift voucher worth USD300 to the most expensive salon in the city, but I told her please no. I would not touch it with a sterilized barge pole!

She was a bit hurt, until I told her that she had to go every 20 days to that saloon, for topping up, and massaging, and facelifts, and face packs and face cleansing and all that jazz, because she had got used to it, and not doing that would make her feel that she was growing old and not looking so good.

So I would rather talk about home remedies and home cures like face packs at home, which you can apply and leave on, while watching TV, or working on your computer.

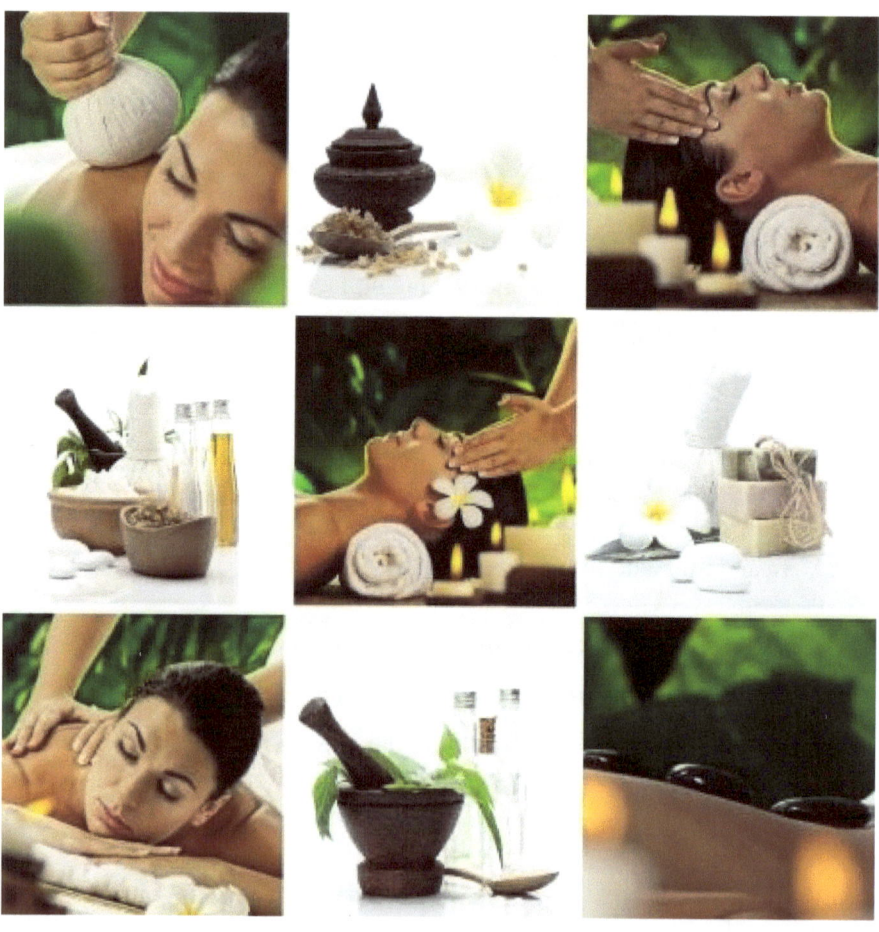

You may want to going for a beauty treatment, once in a Bluemoon, just to indulge yourself, but if the oils are lanolin based, you may find yourself suffering from an acne outbreak.

Each face pack is best applied upon the squeaky clean face. It should be wet and applied from chin to forehead. Make sure that when it is dry you do not rub it off because your facial skin is very delicate.

Relax as much as possible and remove the pack with cotton and warm water, rubbing in circular motions.

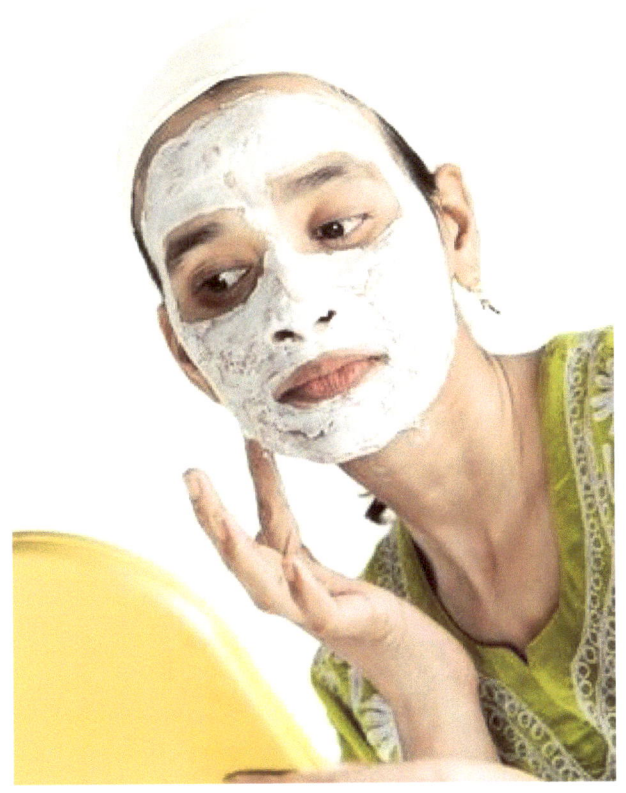

Face Packs and Scrubs

What is the difference between a face pack and a scrub? A scrub is a natural face pack made up of an oil along with a grainy substance like oatmeal, gram flour, or even bran. Face packs are also naturally, but they are more liquid inconsistency. In fact face packs can be made up of any natural substance, for example, take one egg, little bit of lemon, some dried almonds, and rub the mixture all over your face. Allow it to dry for 20 minutes, and you are going to look younger and cleaner looking in a positive way.

Oily Skin

Many times, your skin may not be greasy, but sometimes it looks terrible, especially before a party. What do you do under such circumstances? This recipe was given to me by one of my colleagues, who was training as a future air hostesses in the aviation school, where I was also a faculty member and a manager.

Before you go out on a special occasion, wash your face very carefully with a soft glycerin soap and after that apply the juice of one tomato all over your face. Allow it to dry, then take an ice cube and rub it all over your face and neck.

When you think that your skin is quite dry, wipe your face with a towel dipped in cold water then apply your party make up. It not only makes you feel fresh and cool, but also gives your face a really beautiful glow.

Tomato juice and pulp is the best natural astringent, which you can use as a natural skin toner and cleanser, instead of expensive branded name astringents.

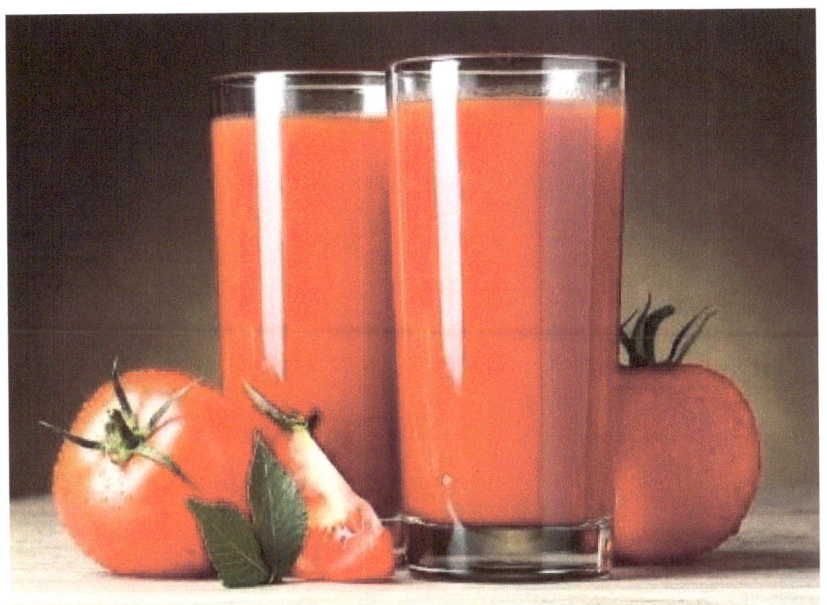

Tomato juice – excellent to drink to detoxify you, and excellent to apply on your face as a toner.

Dry skin

These normally occur when your body is suffering from dehydration. So remember to drink lots of water every day to keep your skin plump and toned.

If you have a very dry skin, you may need to cleanse it with a special facemask. Take 4 teaspoons full of glycerin, 2 teaspoons full of rosewater, a few drops of lemon juice, and two spoons of cooked oatmeal.

Make this into a paste, and spread it all over your face after you have opened up the pores by placing a towel dipped in hot water upon your skin.

After this paste dries up, remove it with hot water as a natural astringent, tomato juice is going to be used to close up the pores, after you allow it to dry on your skin, wash it off and then rub a cube of ice all over your face.

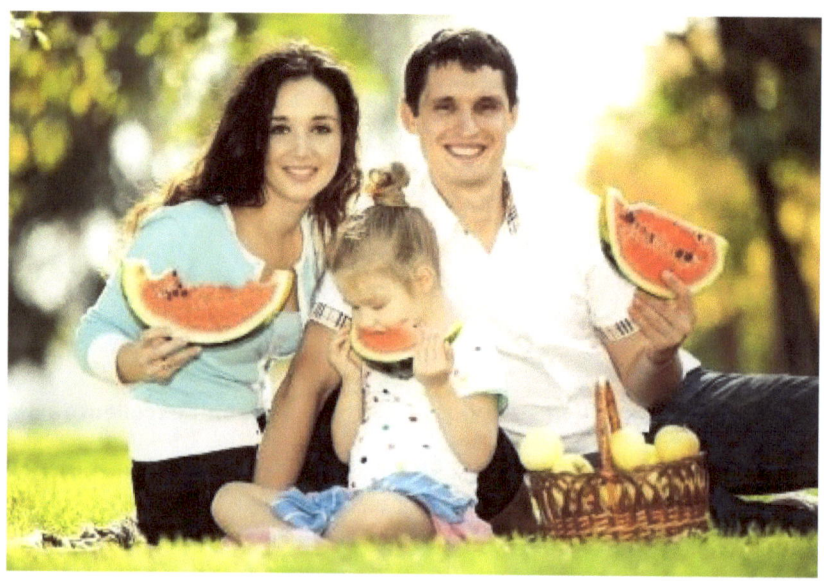

Watermelon juice is excellent for your skin. Just rub the skin against your face, neck, and arms, your skin will be moisturized instantly.

Normal skin

People are very surprised when I tell them that I have not used any soap on my face since I was at college. That was because the soft Pears glycerin soap, which I used to use became temporary unavailable. So I began to look for other natural resorts in order to clean my skin.

This was a mixture of Fuller's Earth, glycerin, and honey. I applied it all over my face, allowed it to dry, and then washed it off, in circular motions with warm water. And this is the cleansing material, I use to this day, without any wrinkles, pimples, or skin problems. [Apart from the chemical burns of course, which are disappearing slowly and steadily and my skin going back to its normal natural tone!]

Here is one beauty secret, which was used by one of the most popular Hollywood stars shooting in a supposedly uncivilized area away from beauty parlors and salons! This was described in Bob Hope's autobiography. Ms. Lollobrigida and he were traveling to their remote destination in a rickety vehicle. It took about eight hours for the journey to take place. The lady just took out a bottle of olive oil calmly, and began massaging her hands, face, neck, and other exposed parts of the body during the drive.

According to him, by the time the drive was over, the bottle was finished!

I of course would not use the whole bottle of olive oil for massaging myself in a journey of eight hours, but she really looked good even when she was in her 60s. However, if you do not have any olive oil at hand, but you do have a medicine box with some Epsom salts for digestion, half your job is done!

However, you will need to have some sort of oil like olive oil or coconut oil at hand for moisturizing your skin. First apply coconut oil all over your face.

Then dissolve 2 tablespoons full of Epsom salts in hot water. Make a cold water bath in a little bowl with ice and 2 tablespoons full of sugar. Now dip a towel in the hot water solution and place it upon your face and neck until it has cooled down. After that, repeat the procedure again with your hot solution – with the Epsom salts dissolved in them – over your face and neck. Do this four times.

After that, switch over to the cold solution. Repeat four times. Continue this treatment for 10 minutes and see how refreshed you feel. Your skin also is going to feel youthful and rejuvenated.

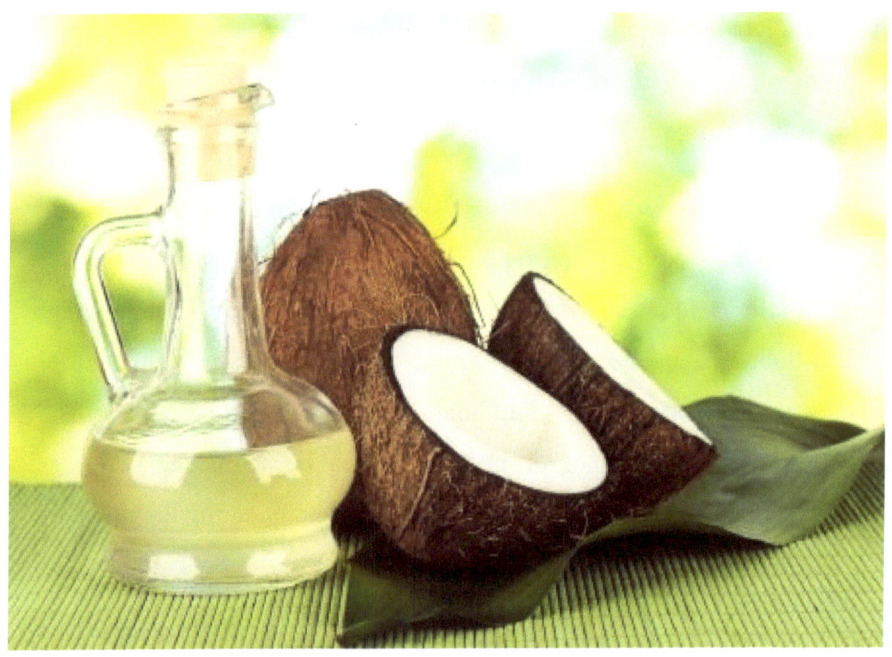

Coconut oil is about the best natural moisturizer you could ever get.

Treating Sunburn

There are many people like I who just cannot resist the elements, sun, rain, and shine. However much they may like it, this creates havoc with their skin, and they turn up all sunburned, which they fondly call a tan.

This tan may be very socially desirable, but it is the worst thing that you could do to your skin. You are burning off the top protective superficial layer of your skin. Bad sunburn can damage your skin irrevocably. Too much exposure to the sun can also cause ultraviolet ray damage, including skin cancer.

My mother was invited by some of her friends to Australia, and she spoke about the daughter of the house, not moving out without slathering anti-suntan cream all over her face and body.

My mother told me that she had never seen so many cases of skin cancer in one place, and that was in the 90s. She said the reason was that the people going to Australia were so thrilled to finally be in a warm place with lots of sun, that they did not know about the damaging effect of the sun on their skin. 20 years later, they were suffering from skin cancer, because they did not bother to protect their skin from the harsh rays or because they thought that it looked so stylish to be tanned and baked in tone.

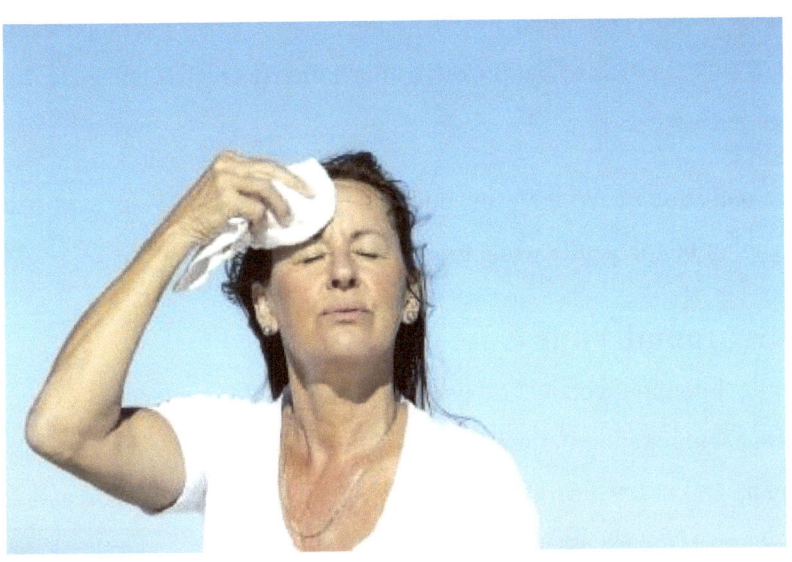

Apart from dehydration, this lady is going to suffer from a severe case of sunburn. You can see the first signs on her cheeks and throat.

So if you have managed to burn yourself, it is time to protect yourself naturally. Try this oil treatment once a week. Take a cloth and make holes in it for your nose, mouth, and eyes. Soak it in a bowl of hot almond oil and leave it on the face for half an hour until it is soaked in, while you relax. It normally takes about this much time to penetrate into the skin.

Remove the excess oil with hot water, after half an hour. This should act as a natural moisturizer against the elements.

Wrinkle Treatment

Taking into consideration the skin texture and age, lines and wrinkles are going to be a part and parcel of growing old dry skin has a tendency of lining faster than a well moisturized skin. So if you are suffering from wrinkles or lines around your eyes, you only have to use a very good muscle oil and only the pads of the fingers with a butterfly touch to massage that oil in that sensitive area.

Work outwards above the eyes, and inwards underneath your eyes because you cannot be too gentle while touching this delicate skin.

Lines around Your Nose and Mouth

Warm a little bit of coconut oil using the two middle fingers of each hand massage with circular motions starting from the corners of the mouth and going up and in towards the nostrils. Continue this for a few moments and then wipe off the excess coconut oil. This procedure is going to be done with your cheeks blown out for 10 minutes every day. This is going to get rid of all the lines around your nose and mouth which are the first sign of aging.

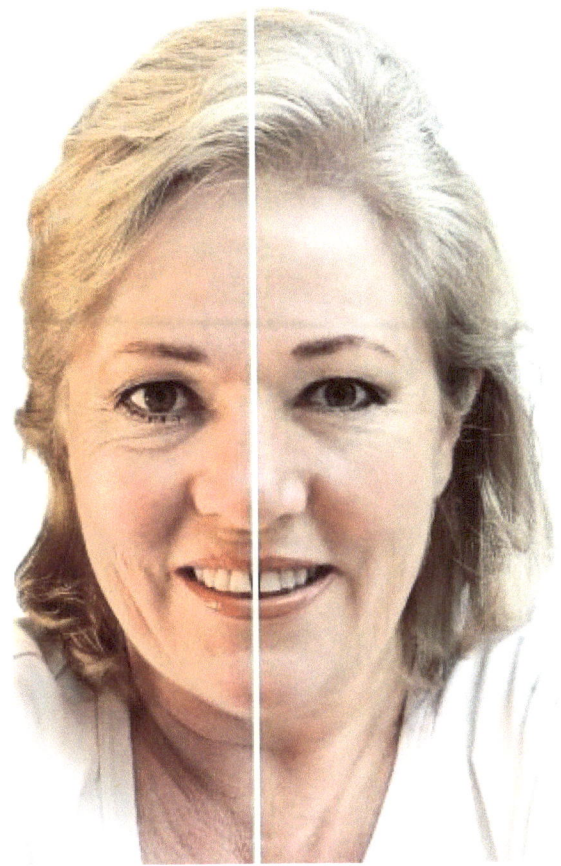

Lines on Your Forehead

These lines on one's forehead are normally removed through expensive and extensive surgical procedures, which are going to put your forehead muscles up to your temples and some other complicated procedure, including your muscles and tissue.

I had these deep lines on my forehead when I was 10 and they definitely never bothered me ever. However, if you are conscious about these lines, which you call the front lines on your forehead. Place your two middle fingers of the right hand at the corner of your left eyebrow.

Use a good oil to moisturize the skin. Massage up and out to the right temple. Do the same for the right side with the left hand.

For horizontal lines, running across your forehead, start in the middle of the forehead and massage with a circular movement along to the sides – the temple region and the upper cheekbones.

Teenage Acne

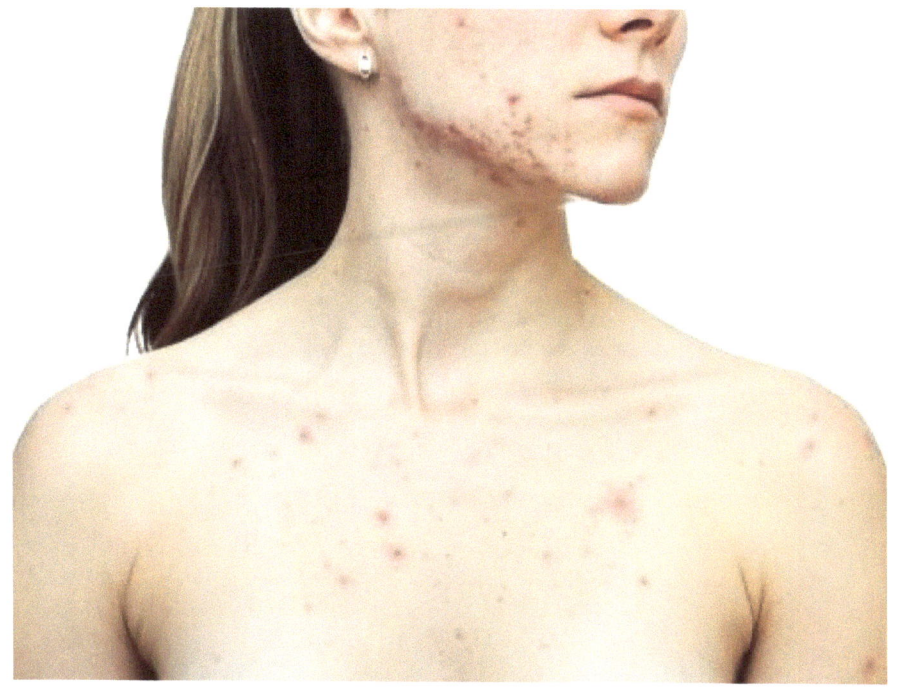

Now this is a terrible case of teenage acne...

Acne is one of the most common of skin ailments which occur during adolescence. Apart from it affecting your appearance, it is also going to have a detrimental effect on your self-confidence. However, teenage acne is one condition which can be cured naturally without leaving any scars.

This is normally associated with excessive hyperactivity of the present oil glands in the skin, and the congestion of pores. The condition of lots of oiliness, is known as seborrhoea. This actually occurs, when the skin glands under the epidermis begin to secrete a large amount of oil. This clogs up all the pores, and causes an infection. This is a general precondition to any formation of pimples, also known as Rosacea and acne on the surface of the skin.

I remember one fine day, when I was the Database Manager at IT FT [Inst. of Tourism and Future Management Trends], more than a decade ago, when one of my colleagues collared me in a very exasperated tone.

What had I done? I had been trying to give my students advice on how to get rid of acne?

Goggle mouthed goldfishes had nothing on me. Actually, this lady had attacked first, before finding out who had given her the advice, but putting one and one together and getting 13, – you are a naturopath, so you must have given this particular student this particular disastrous advice, – and after I had yelled an indignant negative, we both went to check up the extent of the disaster.

This young boy had ground some cloves of raw garlic and applied them all over the affected area. Ouch! That area was now raw, blistered, and red. So never ever try applying anything on the sensitive skin of your face, hoping against hope that the pimples are going to go away.

When I asked him who had given him such a disastrous advice – in the hearing of K, who still was half inclined to believe that I had given him this remedy – he told me that all the girls he knew treated their acne in this manner. After I had stopped shuddering, I immediately told them to stop doing that, because the proof of the pudding was in the eating and right in front of them!

Appearance of Acne

Acne normally appears on your back, face, shoulders and chest. The reason is that the oil glands are more active in these particular areas and also, the hair follicles are always more in quantity in these particular parts of your body.

Symptoms of Acne

Acne normally breaks out in large skin pores that are visible, clusters of little red infected bumps just breaking out on your skin, inflamed whiteheads, and blackheads. Apart from that, your skin is also going to be quite oily.

So how does this acne form?

Formation of Skin Pimples and Acnes

1. Healthy follicle
Sebaceous duct
gland

2. Duct clogged by dead cells, sebum starts accumulate

4. Follicle ruptures, pustule with fluid formed, - acnes

3. Bacterial infection, inflammation triggered, - pimple

Researchers have shown that the activity in the function of the oil glands is normally controlled by androgen, present in your body. This is a male hormone, but it is present both in women and in men in different proportions. That is why both of them are affected by acne. When the androgen levels due to the hyperactivity of the adrenal gland and in case of women, the ovaries, rise, it is going to cause an over activity in the oil glands.

This is going to worsen the skin condition which may be oily already. And this is going to encourage the formation of acne.

Bacterial Infections

There are two main types of bacteria, which are present all over the surface of your skin. Apart from that, there is also a fungus, which is a yeast type of fungus. These are pretty harmless, and noneffective, when they are confronted with normal skin. However, the moment they are confronted with oily skin, they begin to proliferate, and infects that skin area.

These harmful bacteria begin to try when there is congestion or blockages in the pores of the skin. It is a low oxygen environment, now in the glands. The triglycerides present are going to be changed chemically into fatty acids. This means that you are going to have whiteheads erupting on your skin.

When the bacterial infection spreads all over the surface of the skin, it turns the appearance of the skin to red patches. This condition is now known as Rosacea.

Types of Rosacea

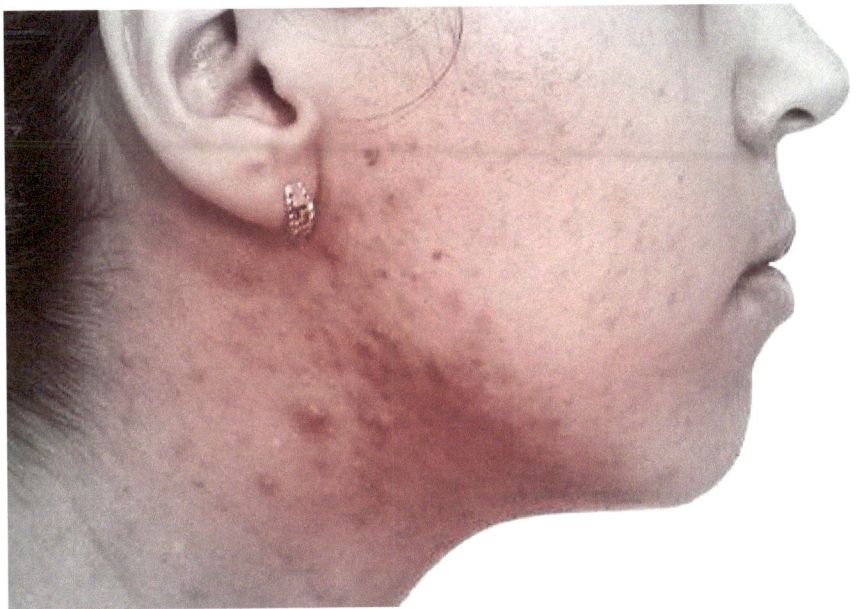

Actually, there are five basic types of Rosacea –

The most common one is the mild type, which is going to affect a large number of teenagers. Most of them are going to have an outbreak, sometimes or the other, during their teenage time, mostly because of hormonal imbalance, and also through a bad diet, lack of exercise, and other factors like a grimy skin and low hygienic standards.

Teenage spots

In a mild outbreak, this particular type of acne is normally known as teenage spots. They are going to last for a few months, and disappear for some time after that, they may appear again. This condition is the easiest to treat.

However, if you are suffering from a severe case of teenage spots, due to improper skincare, which has increased the severity of the condition, now you are going to be suffering from moderate acne.

Moderate acne

Moderate acne is known as acne vulgaris. In about 10% of the cases, if you are suffering from mild acne, the condition is going to worsen due to the prolonged existence of severe oily skin and acne. The number and concentration of the red infected areas and the whiteheads are going to increase. Also, a large number of papules are going to develop.

This is a time when the affected spots are going to turned red. That is because the blood vessels have ruptured.

Generally, this type of acne is not so volatile when you reach your 20s because the spots are going to clear up, as your hormone levels settled down to normal and that of an adult again.

Chronic acne

This is fortunately a rare condition. In this, the red acne spots are more in number, larger in size, painful to touch, and infected.

Under such a circumstance, the entire shoulders' area, back, and the whole face is going to be affected by the acne spots. It is going to take more time to cure this particular ailment. Also, it is possible that this severe outbreak is going to leave scars.

Pickers Acne

This is a condition, when the central part of the spot is going to be covered by a scab. It looks raw. It is not like the tip of a pimple. This is because the spot has been scratched and picked frequently.

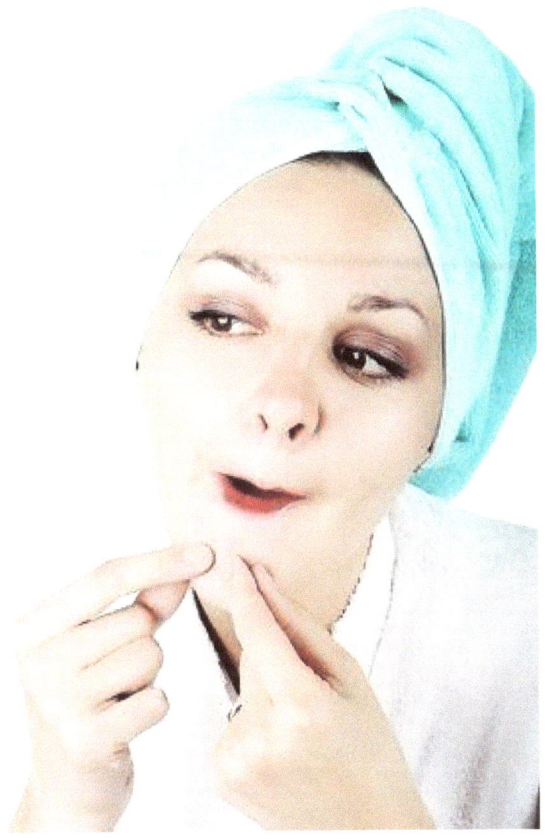

The spots are not very obvious, but they make the person feel fidgety and uncomfortable.

Fringe and Cosmetic Acne

This normally occurs on the forehead area and is mostly due to the excessive grease and oil which clogs up the hair follicles. This happens if you have been applying a lot of grease and oil to your scalp, and also if you are suffering from dandruff.

Aggravation of Acne

There are many factors which are going to aggravate your acne condition. This is going to include picking and constant touching of the affected area.

At college, I remember one of my friends who suffered from a very bad case of acne. You could not get her to stop looking at the nearest mirror, and then wailing over her acne condition and then trying to press the infection out of the infected area. Apart from this activity looking disgusting to the onlookers, it made certain, that the three years we were there, she never had a clear skin.

I saw her a decade later and she was the only adult of our once – classmates group, who had acne scars, and a terrible skin condition. But nobody could teach her not to keep away from the acne, and applying pressure, and picking at those affected spots.

Also, remember never to wear tight sweat bands, if you are suffering from fringe acne. This is going to heighten the risk of scarring.

Vitamin B12 deficiency is another reason why people who suffer from anemia, particularly women may suffer from an acne condition for that you have to increase your dosage of vitamin B12.

Researchers believe that foods which are rich in iodine and drugs, like asthma and cold remedies which contain fluorides, bromides, and iodides are capable of aggravating your acne condition. So if you are suffering from acne, you may want to stop eating spinach and stop brushing your teeth with toothpaste which has fluorides in it.

Also, I remember one of my students applying toothpaste upon her acne because she thought that that was the easiest way in which she could get that condition to dry up. It did not help her at all. In fact, it flared up. Why, that was because her toothpaste was full of fluorides!

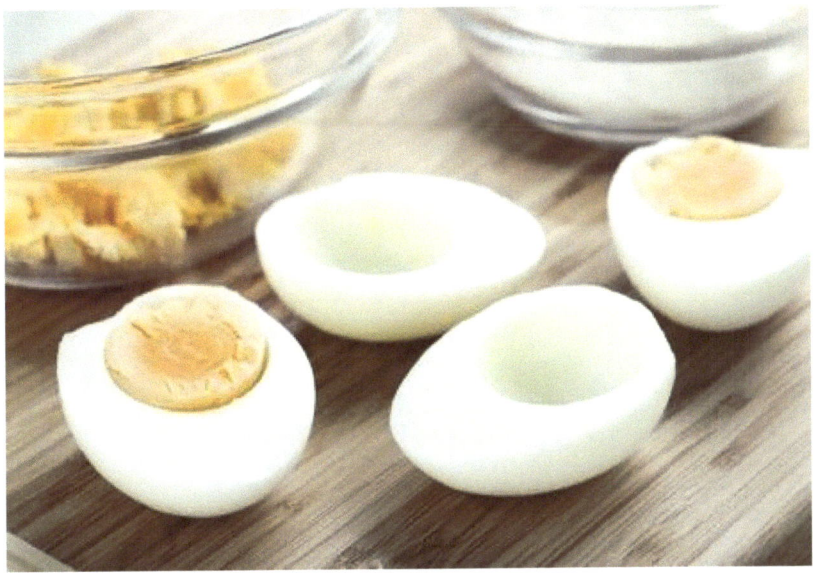

Eggs are an excellent source of vitamin B12.

Let me tell you another amusing incident. I once saw a cook in a restaurant, who stood in front of the fryer, day in day out. The moment he used to enter his kitchen, he covered his face with a piece of cloth, and then began frying the day's meals. When I asked him why he did that, he said that frying at high heat meant frying grease. It would aggravate his acne condition. I think that the cook had something there.

Hot and humid weather is also conducive to acne, because that is the time, when bacteria and fungi flourish on a skin surface. Especially when it is sweaty and wet all the time.

So remember, if you have an acne condition, and the weather turns humid, have some tissues always ready at hand to blot up that excess sweat and prevent the acne condition from worsening.

Lots of water is not only going to cure up any possible skin condition, but it is also going to keep you well hydrated in the summer.

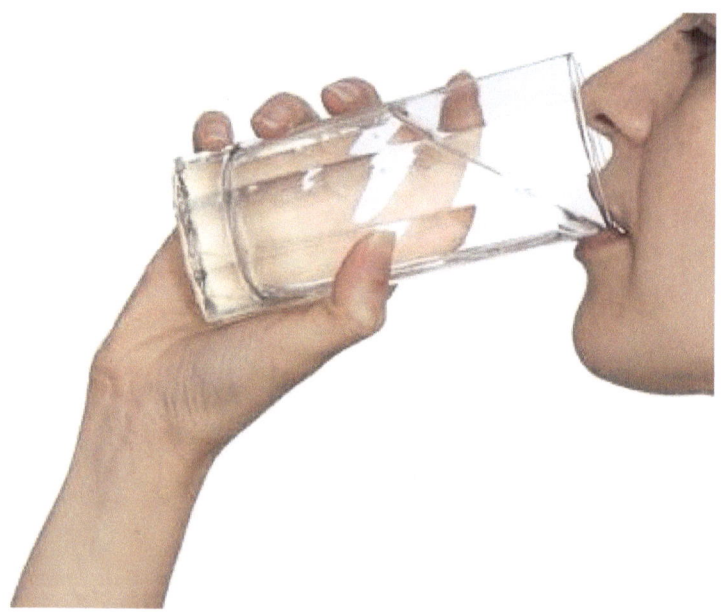

Also, using plenty of lanolin based cosmetics and other cosmetics, which have lots of derivatives of oils and fatty acids are not recommended, because they are going to be potent acne stimulants. Believe it or not, vanishing creams, which are so popular to get rid of spots are quite capable of causing a flare of your acne condition.

Also, if you are suffering from stress and tension, it is going to aggravate your acne condition and then you are going to be stressed out, because you do not feel good with acne spots all over your face. And that is going to cause even more stress. So this can be considered to be a really vicious circle.

This is a time when you have to look for natural treatment or going to a dermatologist. Do not run to the dermatologist, at the slightest flare of acne. This should be done only in chronic cases. If you really want to take the help of a dermatologist, where he is going to treat you with skincare treatment and medical drug treatment, remember to consult an experienced and qualified skincare expert dermatologist.

Remember that such qualified professionals are going to suggest drugs for oral consumption and local application.

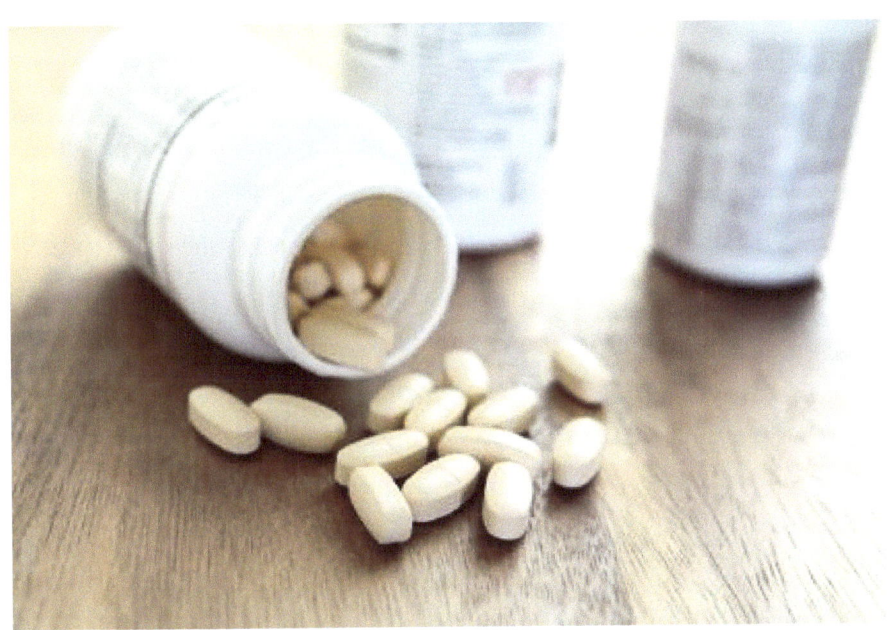

Local drug treatments can be found in over the counter remedies. Some of them are made up of benzyl peroxide. They are either in lotion form or in gel form. Some of them are really strong so remember to use them in very small quantities, if you are applying them on your tender facial skin.

Benzyl peroxide helps to get rid of bacteria. It also releases the necessary oxygen, which helps in healing the anaerobic bacteria.

In a modest case, you can just apply a very thin layer, but if the acne is stubborn, your doctor may prescribe two applications per day.

Do not think that applying a thick layer of a lotion or a cream is going to help get rid of the acne condition quicker. If you are going on the principle of the more you put on, the faster the condition is going to disappear, well, it does not work that way. Instead, you may find yourself suffering from other out break, because you have clogged the pores of your skin with oily ointment.

There are plenty of sulfur drug preparations also available in the market today and most of them are over the counter. They dislodge and lose in the blackheads from the skin pores that is because they cause the skin to peel. So this in itself should tell you how powerful these sulfur based drugs are because they peel off the top layer of your epidermis on application.

Oral Drug Treatments

Your doctor may possibly recommend antibiotics to you, like tetracycline, which normally does not have any side effects. It is supposed to be a safe drug. But I do not really go in for drugs as an advice. However, if you have been advised tetracycline for an oral drug treatment, avoid exposure to the sun. That is because this particular drug causes a photosensitive reaction.

Skincare Routine

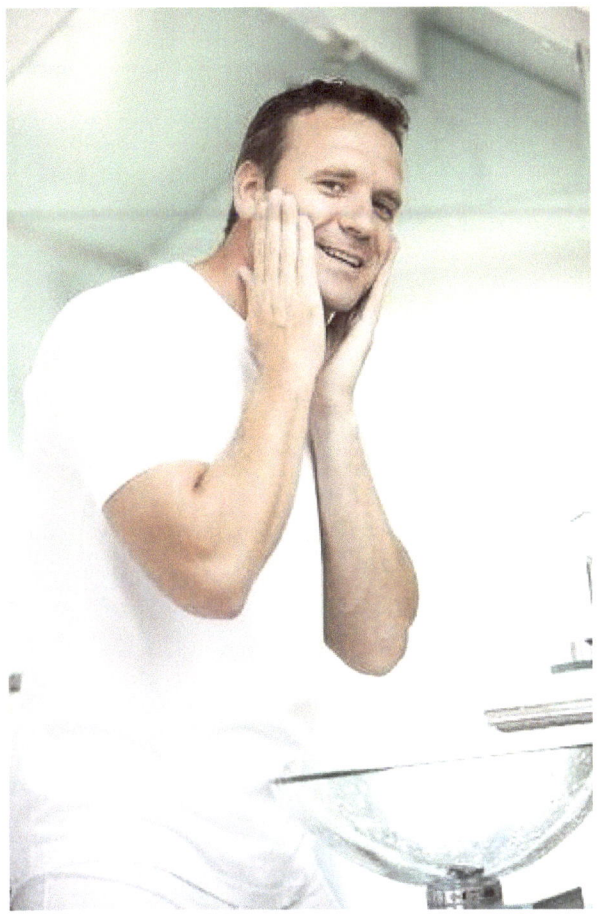

This applies to men too!

People suffering from acne have to make sure that they do not do anything, which can aggravate the condition. Whenever you are cleaning your skin, you need to wash your hands really thoroughly with warm water and wash your skin with a prescribed, medicated, or antiseptic soap. Choose a light liquid cleanser and apply it all over your skin, to get rid of the oiliness.

Rinse thoroughly with clear running water. Pat and dry with a clean, soft towel.

Saturated a pad of cotton with an astringent. I would suggest tomato juice, in which you have added a little bit of water. Even though doctors are going to prescribe medicated lotions for you. Gently press over the entire face and then rinse with cold water. This is going to freshen your skin, reduce oiliness and refine the skin texture.

If you find that area itchy, try soothing it by applying calamine lotion on it, to which you have added a drop of clove oil or mint oil. These are wonderfully refreshing.

At midday, you are going to repeat the treatment you did in the morning. Clean with astringent, medicated lotion/tomato juice, and reapply the medicated cream on the blemishes.

At nighttime, repeat the morning treatment and apply a proper moisturizing lotion on dry areas. These moisturizing lotions may be prescribed to you by the Doctor, but I am going to give you natural healing prescriptions and remedies further on.

Twice a week, you are going to deep cleanse with a friction wash, to control blackheads wet the face with warm water. Take a teaspoonful of cleansing granules into your palm. Add just enough of water to work into a creamy foam. Apply this form to your face with your fingertips. Concentrate on the areas of excessive oiliness and on your blackheads. Massage gently for a few seconds and rinse thoroughly.

Acne tips

Avoid makeup products, creams and ointments, which are lanolin based or oil-based. Do not use any beauty soaps and moisturizers. Avoid eating oily food in your diet and remember to consult a dermatologist if you find yourself suffering from a chronic case of acne.

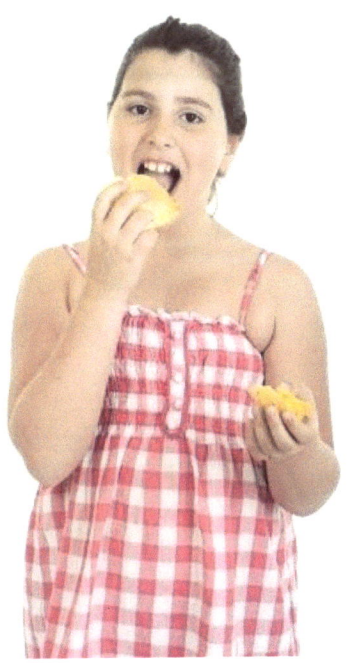

Too much oily food, means acne in the future.

Here are some homemade remedies, which can help cure you.

Apply milk of magnesia on the affected region. Leave it for 10 minutes and then rinse off with warm water.

Make a face pack of 2 teaspoons full of egg white, one teaspoonful of calamine lotion, one teaspoonful of honey, and two cloves of crushed garlic. [Here, the garlic's strong properties are going to be kept in check with the calamine lotion, and the egg white.] Leave this on your face and the affected areas for 20 minutes then rinse off with warm water.

Moisturizer

Make a natural moisturizer with a bottle of rosewater, one fourth teaspoonful of vinegar, five drops of glycerin, and two drops of camphor. This not only dries up your condition, but restores the pH balance of the skin. Also, the rosewater is going to prevent the skin from scarring.

Drying of the pimples can be done by dabbing them with spirit of camphor. This is available at your local drugstore. Keep applying until the pimples dry up. It may sting a little but it is going to check the infection.

Tightening the Pores

The scars are going to be lightened with an icepack used regularly upon the affected area. Wrap ice cubes in a bit of cloth or cotton and apply to the affected area. These are going to help in reducing the enlarged pores.

If you suffer from scarring, here is a natural remedy, which has to be done, when you do not have clothes around, because turmeric stains clothes and skin. Just take one teaspoonful of turmeric powder and put it in milk to make a paste. Apply it all over the affected area. Leave on for 20 minutes and then slowly scrub that off with the tips of your fingers and warm water.

Do this for 15 days, and you are going to see a healthy growth of normal skin. For chronic cases, you may find yourself having to do this for about one month.

I normally get rid of any scars, before my bath, so I do not have to bother about my clothes being stained. This is an excellent timeworn remedy to get rid of scar tissue of any kind. Deep scar tissue is going to take anywhere between 3 to 4 months.

All remaining vestiges of turmeric can be removed with a hot water bath and scrubbing with the loofah.

Conclusion

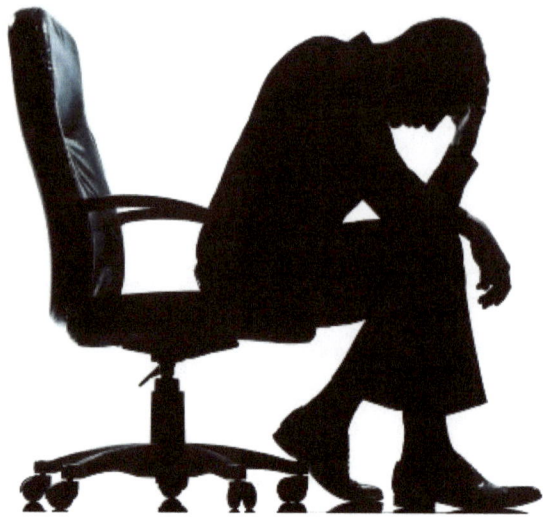

A case of serious acne can sap your self-confidence and make you feel depressed and stressed out.

This book has given you plenty of useful information on how you can keep your skin healthy and looking ageless. Also, it has given you solutions for tackling teenage acne. When there is so much information around you, right at your fingertips, there is absolutely no reason why you should suffer from this tiresome skin condition.

Forget about being depressed. Instead, follow the tips given here and skincare routines properly and then you can face the world with boldness and with confidence.

Live Long and Prosper!

Author Bio

Dueep Jyot Singh is a Management and IT Professional who managed to gather Postgraduate qualifications in Management and English and Degrees in Science, French and Education while pursuing different enjoyable career options like being an hospital administrator, IT,SEO and HRD Database Manager/ trainer, movie , radio and TV scriptwriter, theatre artiste and public speaker, lecturer in French, Marketing and Advertising, ex-Editor of Hearts On Fire (now known as Solstice) Books Missouri USA, advice columnist and cartoonist, publisher and Aviation School trainer, ex-moderator on Medico.in, banker, student councilor ,travelogue writer ... among other things!

One fine morning, she decided that she had enough of killing herself by Degrees and went back to her first love -- writing. It's more enjoyable! She already has 48 published academic and 14 fiction- in- different- genre books under her belt.

When she is not designing websites or making Graphic design illustrations for clients , she is browsing through old bookshops hunting for treasures, of which she has an enviable collection – including R.L. Stevenson, O.Henry, Dornford Yates, Maurice Walsh, De Maupassant, Victor Hugo, Sapper, C.N. Williamson, "Bartimeus" and the crown of her collection- Dickens "The Old Curiosity Shop," and "Martin Chuzzlewit" and so on… Just call her "Renaissance Woman" - collecting herbal remedies, acting like Universal Helping Hand/Agony Aunt, or escaping to her dear mountains for a bit of exploring, collecting herbs and plants, and trekking.

Check out some of the other JD-Biz Publishing books

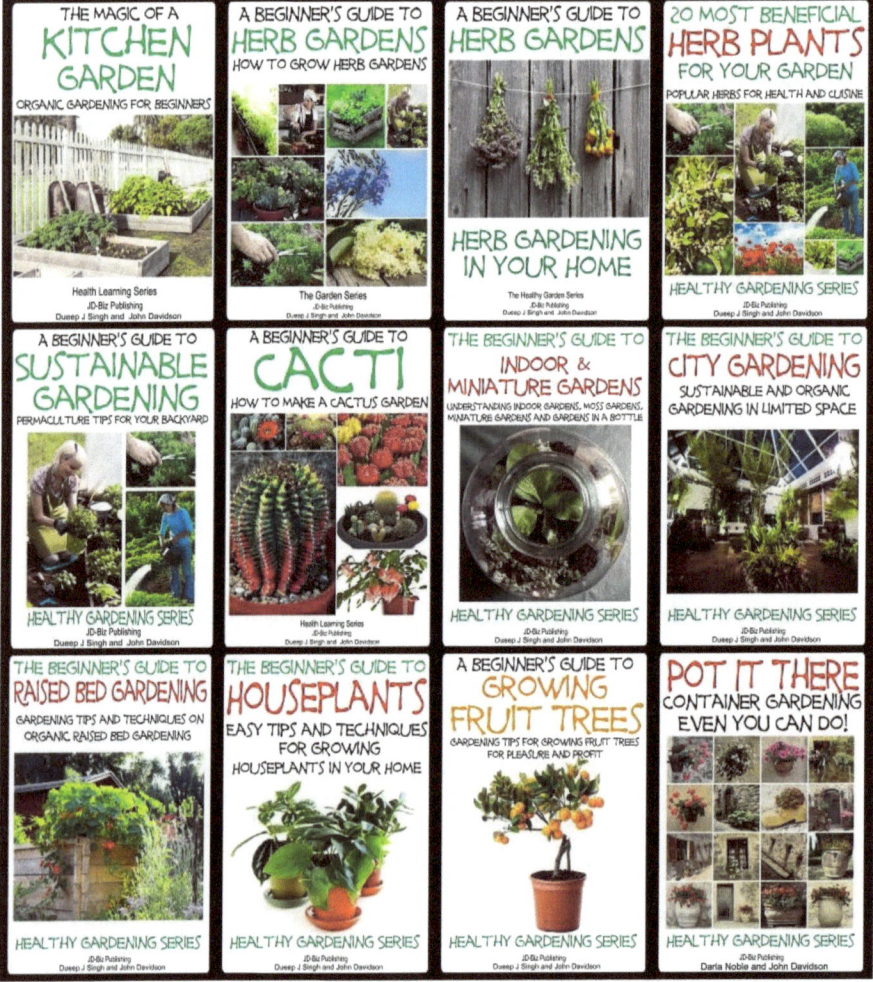

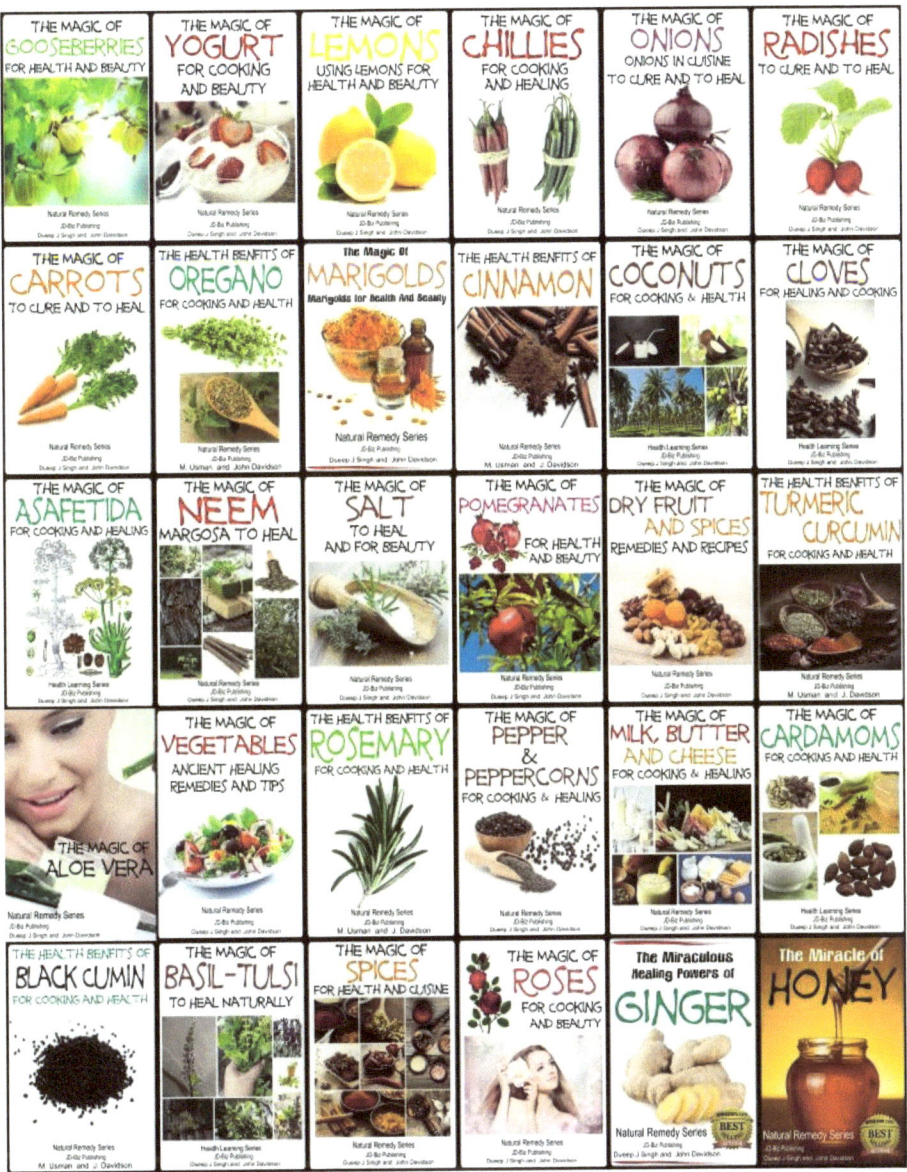

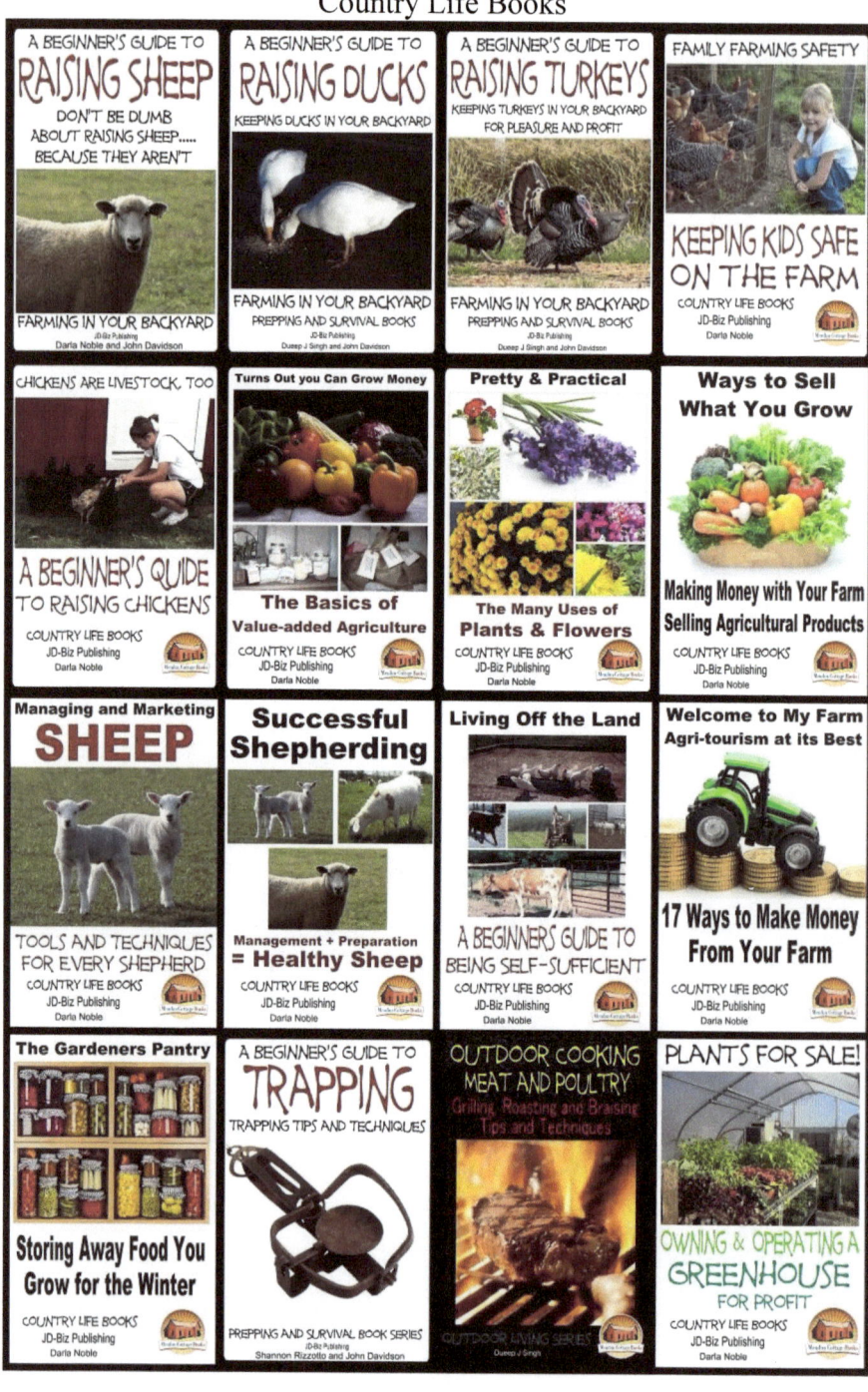

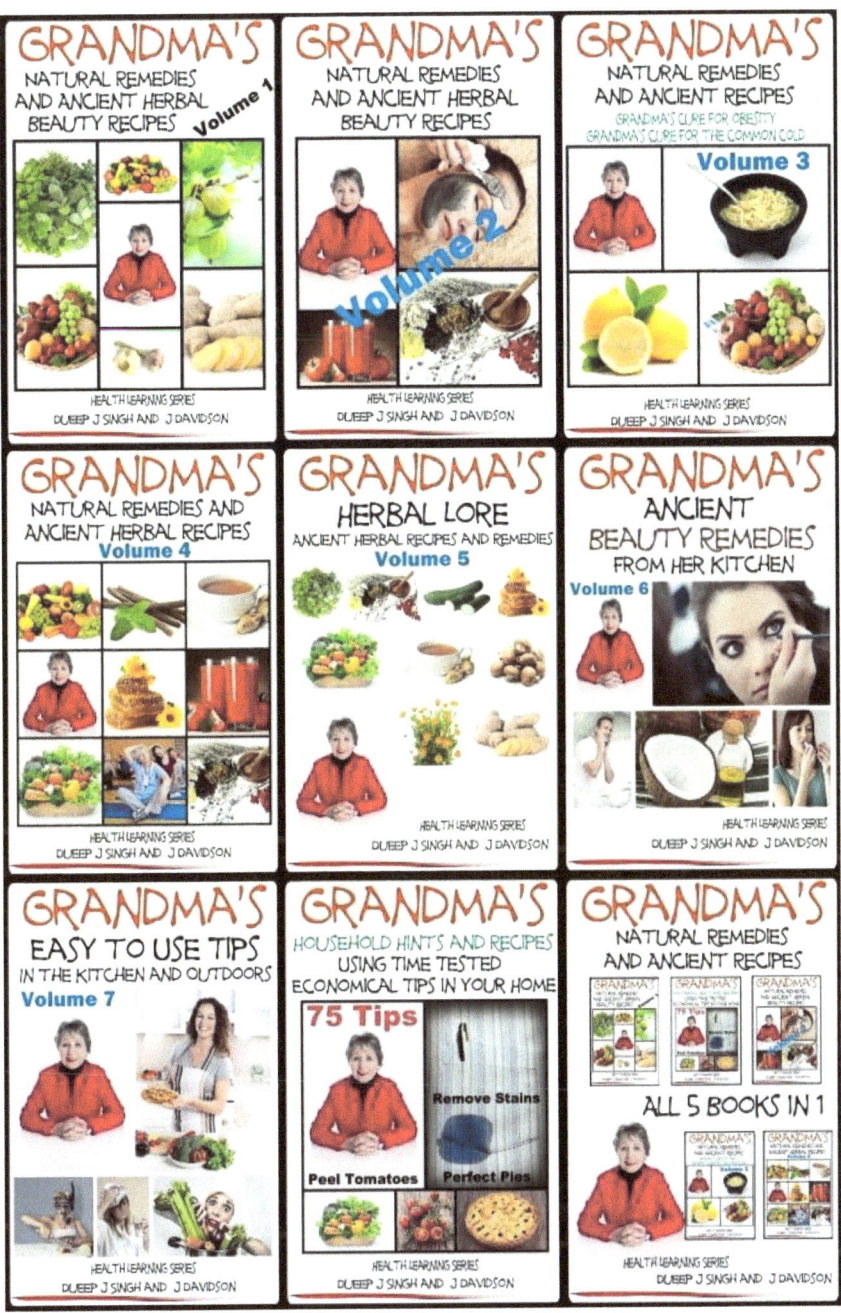

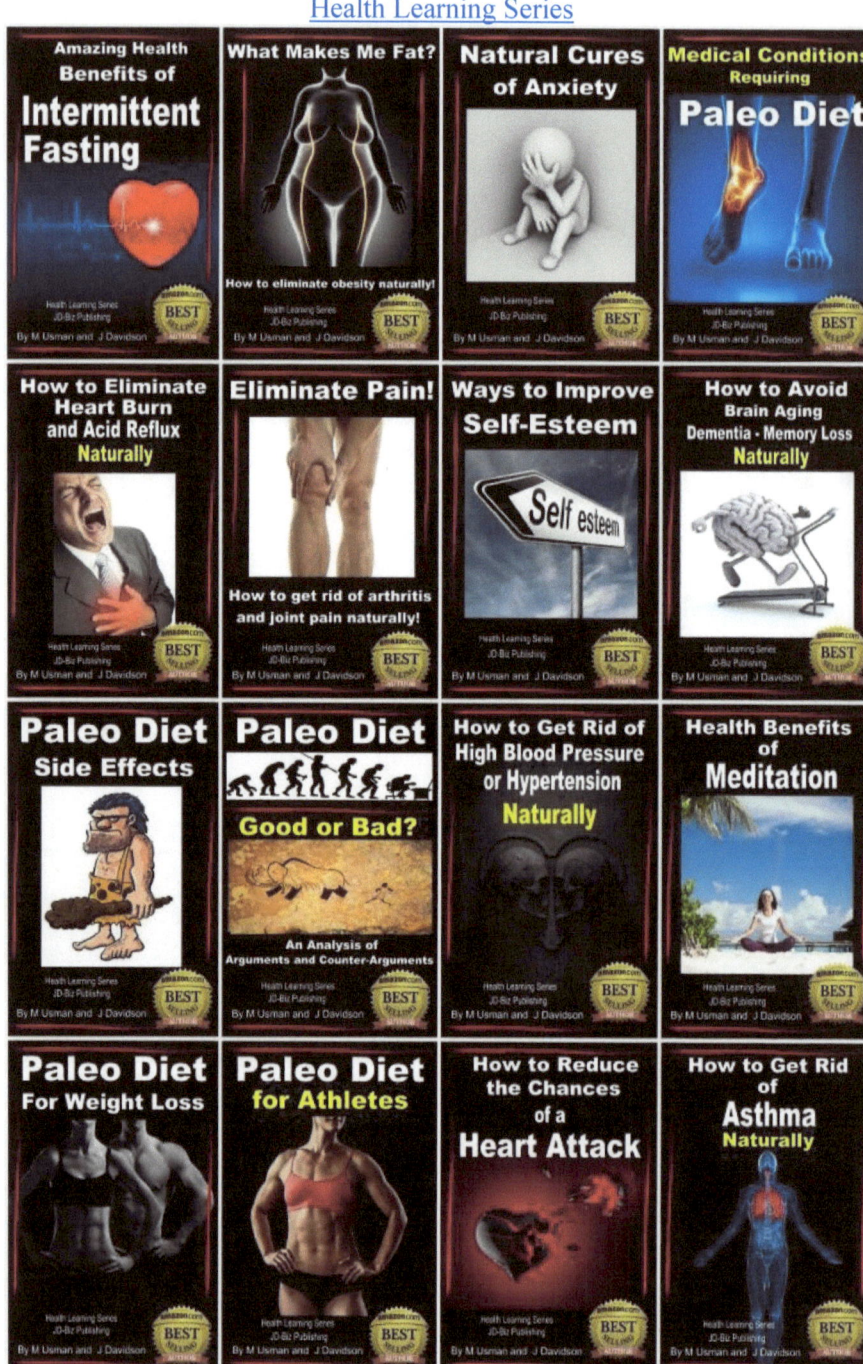

Amazing Animal Book Series

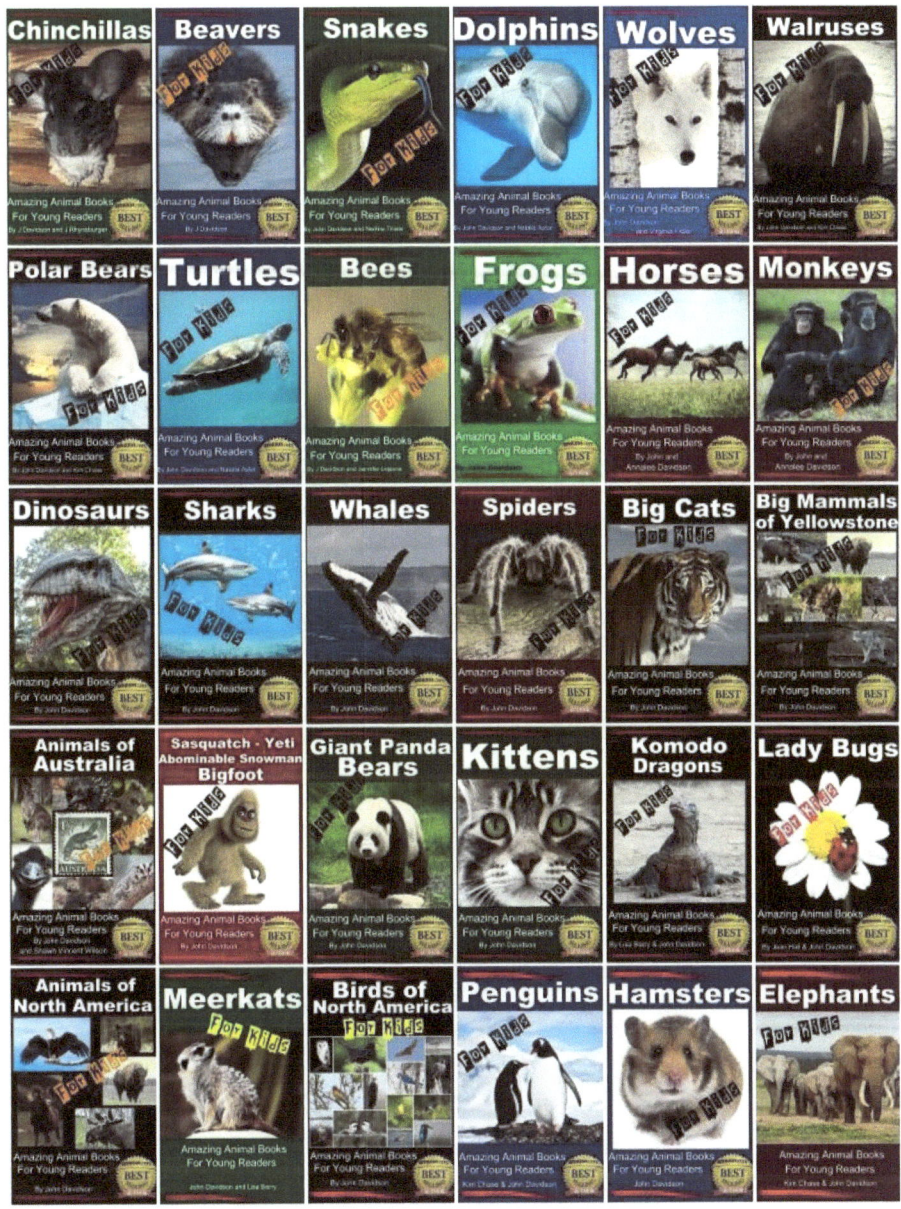

Learn To Draw Series

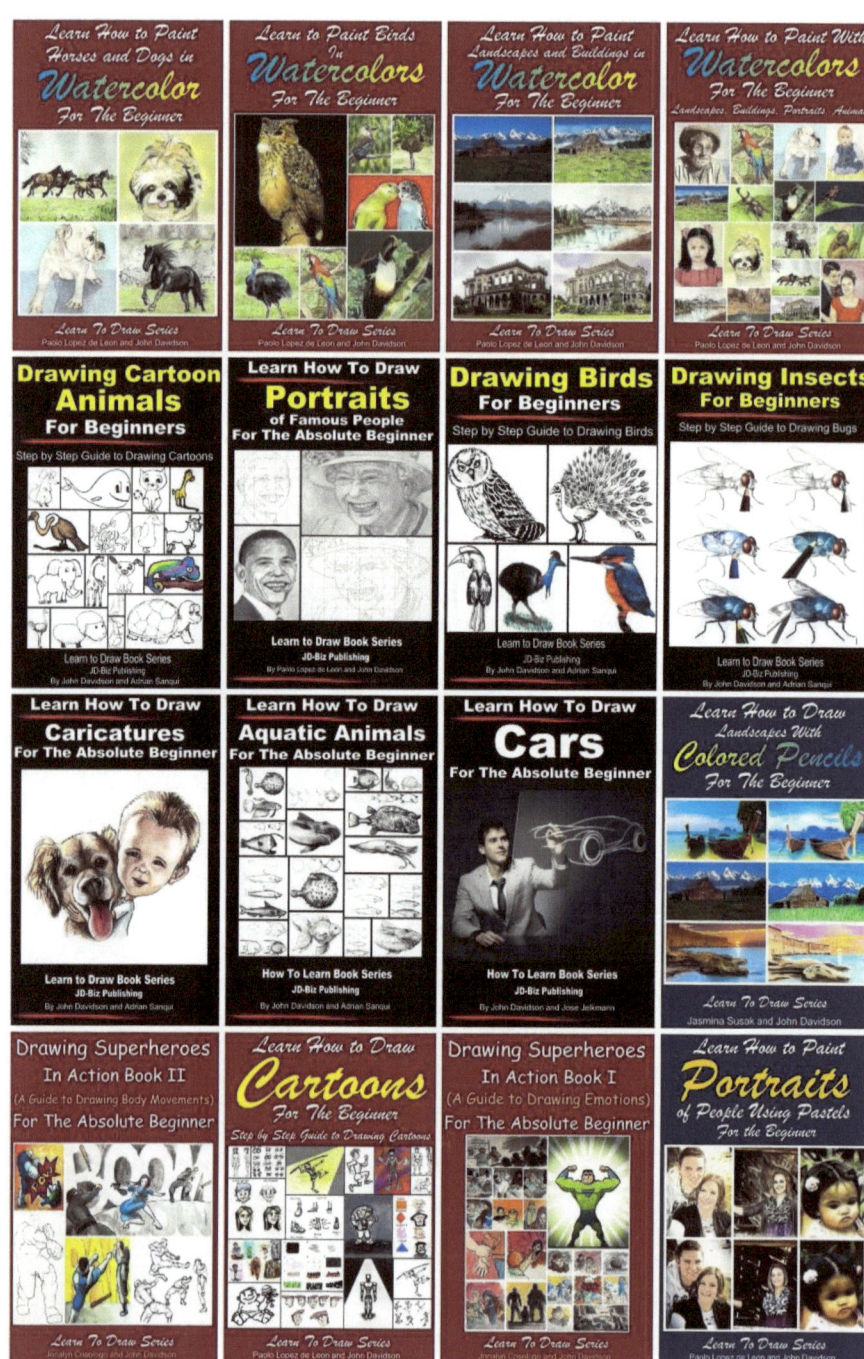

How to Build and Plan Books

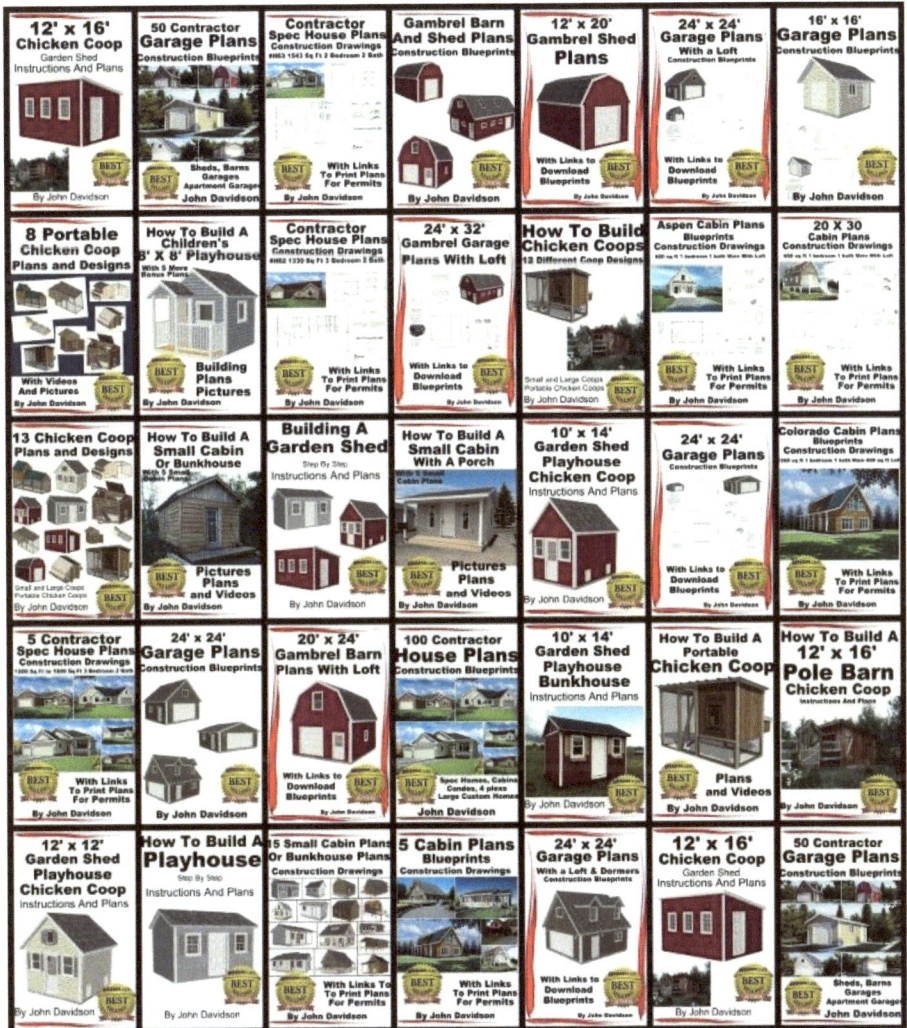

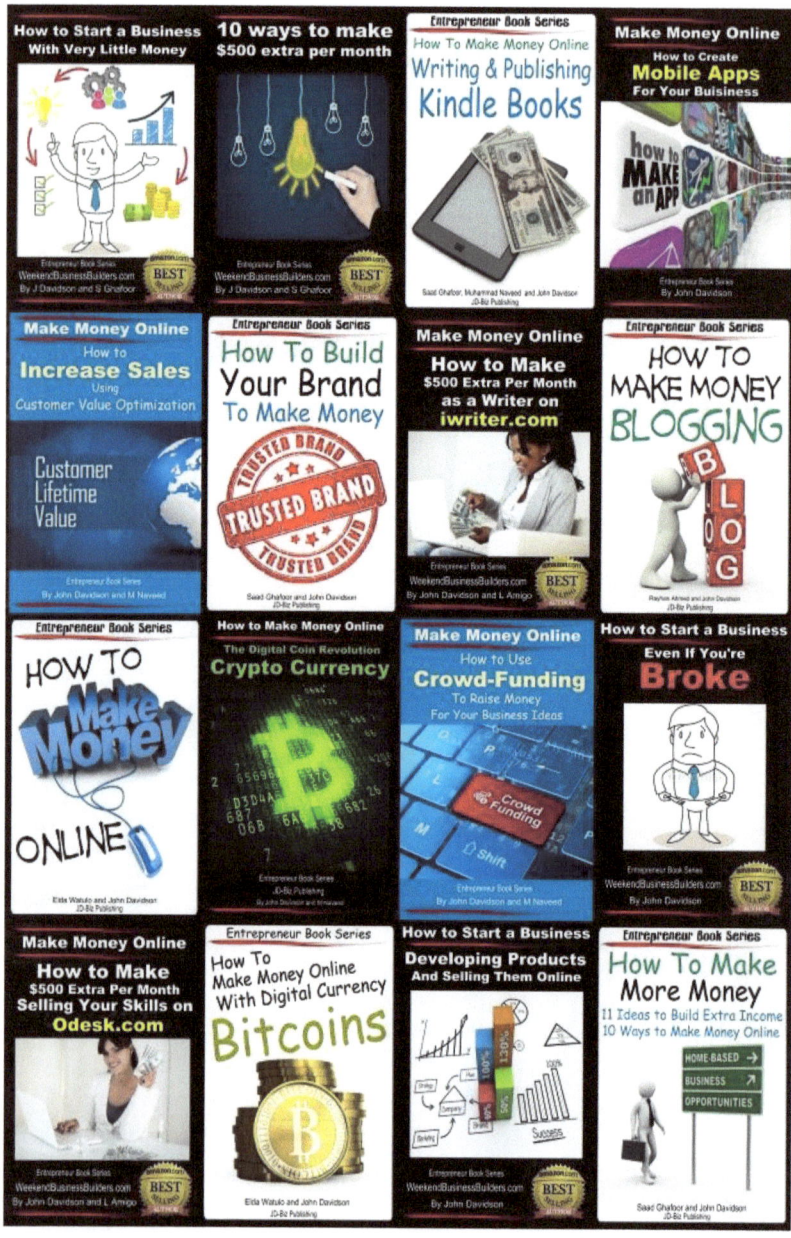

Our books are available at

1. Amazon.com

2. Barnes and Noble

3. Itunes

4. Kobo

5. Smashwords

6. Google Play Books

Download Free Books!

http://MendonCottageBooks.com

Publisher

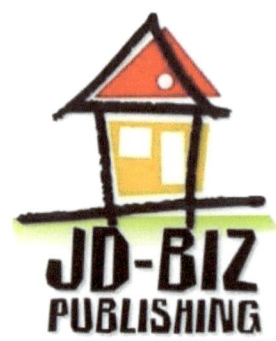

JD-Biz Corp

P O Box 374

Mendon, Utah 84325

http://www.jd-biz.com/

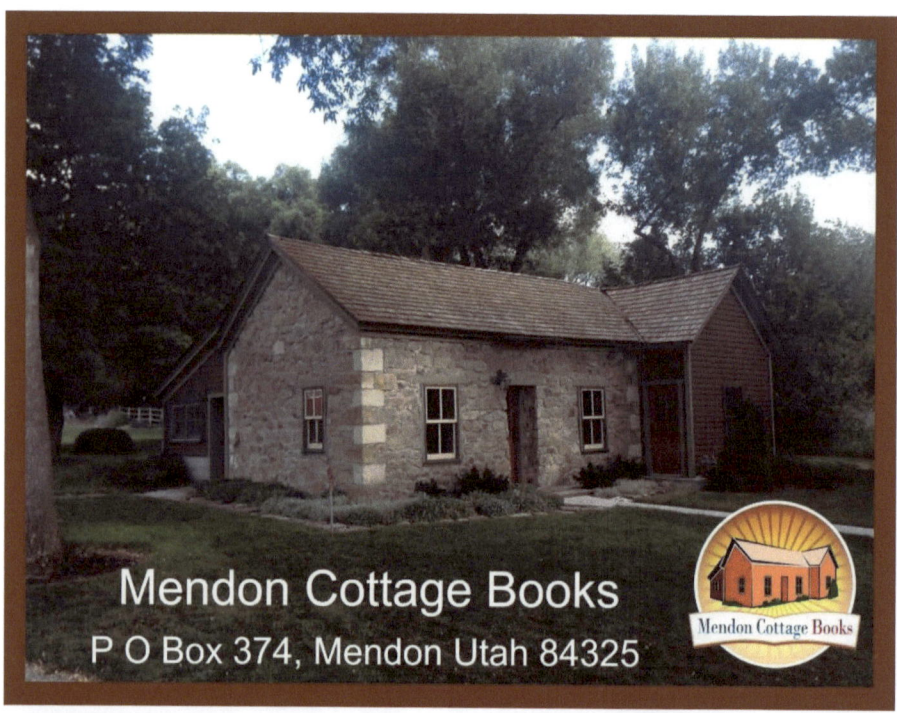

www.ingramcontent.com/pod-product-compliance
Lightning Source LLC
Chambersburg PA
CBHW050830290526
45792CB00001B/339